Menopause Maggie
Change The Change
Naturally

By Kathleen Morr

Copyright Kathleen Morris 2016
Createspace Edition
ISBN 978-1-927828-37-3

Dedication

This book is dedicated to all my friends in the Menopause Maggie Facebook group.

Health Disclaimer

I am not a healthcare professional, and I do not profess to be one. Any information in this book is meant to be for educational purposes only. Personal opinions and experiences expressed by this author, are not to be taken as medical advice, and to be used at your own risk. This author is not responsible for anyone choosing to seek natural therapies. It cannot be used to replace professional medical advice. Please consult your doctor or naturopath concerning the information in this book.

Table of Contents

Introduction

I started the Menopause Maggie Facebook group, as a way for women all over the world, to connect during one of the most difficult transitions we will ever face. Menopause. It's almost like a dirty word. Nobody wants to talk about it, and when the word comes up in conversation, most people make a joke. I'm here to tell you that it is not a joke, and it is not by any means easy.

Let me tell you a little bit about myself before going any further. I knew nothing about menopause. It's not information mothers easily pass down to their daughters. If you are one of the exceptions, I say bravo to you. I don't know what it is about this *change* that makes us keep secrets about it. Perhaps it's because it's an embarrassing subject. We women talk amongst ourselves about menstruation, and PMS, but not a lot. For some reason, bodily functions are taboo.

For me personally, I was embarrassed about even saying the word *period* when I was a young teenager. I didn't want to *become a woman*, because I was more of a tomboy. I wore double sweatshirts to cover my growing breasts, and was terribly uncomfortable in my own skin. When I got my period for the first time, I thought I was dying. I cried and thought it was the end of the world. I couldn't even tell my best friend that I had beaten her to womanhood. I remember briefly talking to my sister about it, and pleading her to call it something other than *period*, because I hated the word so much.

So, why do we women have a difficult time talking about the bodies God gave us? Not all women I guess, but most. The general consensus is to keep a closed lip whenever dealing with menstruation issues, like painful periods, PMS, bloating, flooding, clotting, irregular cycles. Am I making you cringe? These words are not easy to write, or even say for most women. All our lives we avoided this topic like the plague, so how can we expect it to be any different when menopause rears its ugly head?

If you didn't like to talk about your period, you most certainly won't like to talk about your menopause. But there is more to the word menopause than meets the eye. It's not just as sudden change in your body. It changes you mentally, physically, and spiritually. It literally turns you into somebody else, and that's not always a good thing. It *can* be, if we women band together to help each other through, but for the most part, we all suffer in silence. After all, we're women. We don't put ourselves first. We've spent a lifetime taking care of others, that we've forgotten to take care of ourselves. Now we *have* to. If we don't, we won't survive the change.

I found these truths at only 47 years old. Menopause hit me hard, and knocked me off my feet before I even knew what was happening. I thought I was way too young, but apparently not. Thinking back, I realized my body was going through what they call perimenopause at around 42. I told my doctor I was feeling hot and sweaty at night, and wondered if I might be heading into menopause, but he just told me I was too young and not to worry about it for a long time.

He was wrong.

I figured out that general practitioners really don't know much about menopause. In fact, they can't even give a clear answer as to what hot flashes are caused from. I learned early on, that doctors don't always know what's best for you in dealing with menopause. Red flags went up so many times when asking questions.

I knew right away that I would never take hormone replacement therapy, or medications for menopausal symptoms. I had a difficult time taking the pill when I was younger, and developed blood clots in my legs, so I knew I never wanted to experiment with any kind of unnatural hormone replacement again. It was just something I stuck with going into this change, and that's just me. I want all you ladies to know, that it is perfectly fine to take whatever you need to take, to get through menopause. Everyone is different. We need to embrace that, and not fight amongst ourselves with natural, versus unnatural therapy, for menopause.

I wanted to write a book about natural remedies, simply because that is my choice. Perhaps one day I will write a book about HRT, or bio identical hormones, and the numerous medications one can take for menopause, for those who choose that pathway. I just want to be clear, that I am not steering anyone into one direction or another. I support all choices. We're all in this together.

So, here I was, 47 years old, and I hadn't had a period in over a year. What on earth was going on? My periods were on and off for several years. Raise your hand if you thought you were pregnant in your mid-forties because of this? Those thoughts crossed my mind, and drove me crazy, even though my husband had a vasectomy. How insane is that? But it happens to us women. All kinds of thoughts go through our minds during this crazy time in our lives. We can make ourselves sick, thinking all sorts of things are going on, like pregnancy, or cancer, simply because we have not had a period in months.

I tell you, I was not prepared for this. And when I did have a period, it was like I was bleeding to death. How lovely is that, especially working full time dealing with flooding issues, which are quite common during perimenopause, and a very early sign that you are headed toward menopause. Another fact I didn't know.

Awareness is the key, and communication is the means by which we empower ourselves through this change. The more we know, the less afraid we are. Knowledge is power! It's the difference between insecurity, and confidence, during this most crucial life-changing event called menopause.

So off I went to a new doctor, telling him that either I'm going crazy with thinking someone like me could be pregnant at my age, or I was sick, and surely going to die. Either way, I told him something strange was going on, because I was getting these night sweats and hot flashes as well. Immediately, he sent me off to a gynecologist.

The gynecologist gave me a thorough exam, and I was somewhat relieved when he set me up for blood work to check my FSH levels. Something else I never knew. What on earth was an FSH level anyway? I quickly learned that it was a follicle-stimulating hormone test, that measures the amount of follicle-stimulating hormone (FSH), in my blood. FSH helps control menstruation, and produces eggs in our ovaries, It's made in our pituitary gland. Who knew?

How could I not know this stuff?

My gynecologist reassured me that I would be just fine. He said the blood work would tell him everything, but just in case, he wanted to give me a pregnancy test, because as we all know women do have *change of life* babies. I was glad he was thorough, but very embarrassed. All I wanted to do was get out of there.

The test results came back, and I can't remember exactly what the number was, but it was a very high FSH level, that indicated full menopause. I remember he chuckled and said, "I know what's been going on. You are in menopause, my dear." I nearly cried in front of him and said, "But that's impossible. I'm only 47. He told me it wasn't impossible. He told me it's quite normal. He told me to try natural remedies for menopausal symptoms if at all possible. If I couldn't, he would prescribe something for me. I nodded my head, and swallowed hard trying to take it all in. The doctor smiled and gathered his papers from the counter and said, "Welcome to your new life."

I drove home with tears in my eyes, and wondered why he would say, "Welcome to your new life." It wasn't a new life. As far as I was concerned, my life was over. I was an old lady, a wrinkled old lady with gray hair and leathery skin. I had lost my youth, my beauty, and my femininity. I was a man.

You may laugh, but the stuff going on in my head at that time was ridiculous. I had nobody to talk to. Nobody I knew was going through menopause at this age. I felt alone and hopeless. I knew I had to do something about it, but what?

At first I did nothing but wallow in my own sorrows. I grew fatter and fatter until I didn't even recognize my reflection in the mirror. And it wasn't because I was scarfing down food left and right. I was eating normally. In fact, I hadn't changed a thing in my diet, yet the scale kept going up. I didn't have any curves anymore, and my waist was getting so thick that I really did look like a man. I remember bawling on the phone with my sister asking, "How big will I get?" I had already gained 50 pounds in a very short time. I would ask my husband and my friends if I looked fat, and they all lied to me. Every single one of them.

Not only had my body changed in size and shape, but I had started to develop some severe health problems. If I kept going with my weight gain, I would soon be battling diabetes and heart disease. I did not want that. I had to do something. I also struggled with debilitating dizzy spells for no apparent reason. Add that to the night sweats and hot flashes, as well as the sleepless nights, and you can see just how miserable I was.

My dizzy spells were so bad that my husband rushed me into emergency one morning, thinking I was having a stroke. I felt like I was really going to die, only to have the emergency physician tell me there was absolutely nothing wrong with me. It was very frustrating. But my shoulders and my muscles ached so badly, that I could barely cope. I didn't know what this was, but I thought if this is menopause, then I'm done for.

I was prescribed many different things for the dizziness, but nothing ever helped. I practically lived on Tylenol for my muscle aches, and even that didn't help. I got so fed up with doctors, that one day I desperately stormed into my local health food store, and asked for a natural muscle relaxant. I was given a bottle of magnesium that would change my life forever.

After only a few days, my dizziness went away for good, and my muscle pain was gone. And that started my journey into natural health, which in turn, brought me back to the woman I once was. Over a period of two years, I lost 50 pounds, got my curves back, and my youthful happy-go-lucky self.

The following chapters explore the numerous natural methods I use to this day, as well as many other popular natural remedies, that have helped millions of women around the world. My hope is to share them with you, so that you too, can reclaim your youth, and become empowered to take control of your own health.

Chapter 1 – Minerals

Magnesium

I want to share God's miracle mineral with you. Magnesium has completely changed my life, and I know it will change yours too.

Magnesium might very well be the best hot flash remedy of all time, and most people don't even consider it. Yet it is what should form the foundation of natural health, in the menopausal woman.

As I said in my introduction, I stumbled upon magnesium accidentally. Most people don't even know they are magnesium deficient. I found out the hard way, that my magnesium levels were so low, causing me to suffer from severe dizziness. This is one of the main symptoms of magnesium deficiency.

As for magnesium's relationship with menopause, it seems quite clear that a multitude of menopause symptoms are identical to magnesium deficiency symptoms. There have been many women who have experimented with magnesium during menopause, only to find the majority of their symptoms disappear after as little as three days. That was all it took to take away my chronic dizziness.

I also wanted to point out, that my dizziness didn't just start at menopause. I had always struggled with some sort of dizziness since I was a young adult. For no apparent reason, the room would start spinning, and there was nothing I could do about it. Doctors didn't know why, and I had seen many. They all said it probably had something to do with my ears, but they never knew for sure. I couldn't see how that could be, because no matter what remedy I tried, I still had dizziness for no reason at all.

I remember after the birth of my second child. The health nurse came over to check on the baby, and I felt so unwell. My dizziness came back with a vengeance, and as I held my newborn in my arms, while the nurse talked to me, the room started spinning. I politely excused myself, ran to the bathroom with baby in arm, and puked in the toilet. It was one of the most embarrassing moments of my life.

The health nurse thought I had mastitis, but I didn't. She couldn't figure out why I would feel so dizzy. I can understand why she thought I had an infection, but as I said it was completely unexplainable.

My dizziness left me, on and off, sometimes for years, but it always came back and I didn't know why. When I started into menopause, I hadn't had the dizziness for a while. It seemed to get worse all of a sudden, way worse than I had ever experienced before in my entire life. I wondered what had triggered it to become so severe.

Menopause did, but why?

All it took was a trip to the health food store, and my first bottle of magnesium, for me to realize I had found the cure for my dizziness. After only three days of taking magnesium citrate, I felt like my old self again. It was truly amazing.

I began to research magnesium, and found that it controls 1300 biological enzymes in the body. Magnesium really is responsible for every function in your system. Simply put, if you don't have magnesium, you die. The less you have, the poorer your health.

Some people are already born with a magnesium deficiency. It is said that magnesium deficiencies may even be passed down in utero. If our mothers had low magnesium, we also may suffer. I really wish I knew this back when I was pregnant with my three kids. They teach you everything else about how to keep your body healthy during pregnancy, but never one single solitary word about magnesium.

Did you know that the highest concentrations of magnesium are found in your heart? Doctors don't even know this stuff. It's incredible. It makes me mad. Even heart transplant recipients know the value of magnesium. I have a friend who had a heart transplant, tell me that they hooked her up to an I.V with pure magnesium, when she was admitted to the ER.

As we age, our magnesium gets lower and lower. What does that say about our hearts? Do we not need this stuff to have a healthy heart? I think so. My heart was one of my main concerns when entering menopause. I had often heard about menopausal women having heart attacks, and that worried me. I was especially worried because heart disease runs in my family, and I also have a heart murmur. It was diagnosed as an innocent murmur, but nevertheless, my irregular heartbeat especially worried me as I entered menopause.

I have also struggled with chest pains my whole life. My doctor always told me it was just muscle cramping around my heart. I never knew whether to believe him or not, but regardless, it happens even when I'm sitting doing nothing. There is a medical term for it, but as I've always stated I am not a doctor so I don't want to go into that part of it. All I know is that along with my innocent heart murmur, I also have some kind of innocent pain in my chest muscles that has nothing to do with a heart attack and doesn't mean I have heart disease. Still, it worried me as I entered menopause.

The more I took magnesium, the healthier my heart felt. I know that sounds odd to say, but it's true. I had these heart palpitations where it seemed like my heartbeat sped up all of a sudden. Another crazy symptom of menopause. If you've ever had this, and I'm sure you have if you're reading this book, then it is one of the scariest symptoms of menopause. It often goes together with a sudden anxiety or doom feeling. I hated it. But it all went away with magnesium.

I still get that doom feeling sometimes that comes on you just before a hot flash, but it's all very mild now. That includes my hot flashes. Magnesium basically calmed me down. And that's understandable since magnesium is actually a muscle relaxant.

After taking magnesium for more than three years, I went to the doctor for a physical. She sent me for heart tests to see the status of my heart murmur. When I sat down with her and asked her about my heart murmur, she looked at the results and said, "What heart murmur?" I gasped.

I believe magnesium has healed my heart murmur. I also believe that magnesium took away my heart muscle pain, because as soon as I started taking magnesium, the heart pain disappeared and didn't come back. Now that's truly amazing!

If magnesium can relax your muscles, it can relax your heart, it can heal your heart, it can take away heart palpitations. Every menopausal woman in the world should be taking magnesium supplements. I can't stress this enough.

I could go on and on about the benefits of magnesium, but I don't have enough room in this book to say anymore. All I do want to say before I go through the types of magnesium, is to send a shout out to

Dr. Carolyn Dean, and Morley Robins, and the Magnesium Advocacy Facebook group. These people, and this group, also changed my life.

Menopause Maggie got started from the Magnesium Advocacy Facebook group. MM is actually a sister group. We work in conjunction with the main group, to help menopausal women specifically. Even though I am not a doctor, and I don't have any classification to help anyone, I felt it necessary to start a Facebook group, where all menopausal women could gather to support each other. So basically, it's a support group for women going through the change, but more importantly, women who have discovered that magnesium is the key during menopause. The premise of the group, is that without magnesium, we would be wrinkled up old birds. Thus, the group's mascot depicts an old magpie with her tongue hanging out. Maggie!

I found Dr. Carolyn Dean through a Google search one day, when researching menopause. and quickly realized that she is the leading MD on magnesium research in the world. She has developed a number of magnesium supplements, that far exceed the current supplements in any health food store. I'll cover some of those below, but for now, I just wanted to mention, that she was my starting point in my magnesium venture. If you ever have a chance to read her website, please do.

Morley Robins is the founder of the Magnesium Advocacy Group, and he too is a leader in magnesium research. His story is quite unique, and one worth checking out. He is also a wellness Coach, and has helped many people. The best place to get a hold of them is through the Magnesium Advocacy Facebook group, but I'd highly recommend going to his website as well.

I briefly wanted to touch on the types of magnesium, even though I am not as informed as Dr. Carolyn Dean, or Morley Robins. I wanted to give you a rundown of the basics anyway. If you want more details, or a more in depth look at the types of magnesium, I would recommend contacting either one of them for more details, or joining the MAG group.

Magnesium Citrate

I didn't know any better when I started taking magnesium citrate. It did the job quite well, but it is a laxative. I just wanted to point that out right away because it will make you have the runs. They say that you have to slowly build up tolerance, but I'm here to tell you that even if you do that, you're still going to have very loose bowel movements.

Don't get me wrong, magnesium citrate is amazing, because any magnesium is amazing, but it doesn't absorb as well as other types of magnesium, because it goes directly to the gut. Some people might have a different experience, but generally speaking, citrate is a laxative, and great for those who need it, but not so great for those who don't.

I used magnesium citrate for a long time before trying other types. It has a special place in my heart because it fixed me. It wasn't until much later, that I decided I didn't want to run to the bathroom so much. I decided to look into other types of magnesium, like the kind that absorbs through the skin. I'll cover that later on, but for now I just wanted to mention how stubborn I was. It's laughable now, but there *are* other types of magnesium you could try, that may work much better.

If you want to keep your costs low and you don't mind taking a laxative every day, magnesium citrate may be for you. Dosages very, but as I said, you have to build up tolerance in your body very slowly with this type of magnesium. I started with two a day and built up from there.

Magnesium Oil

Anything that can be absorbed by the skin, is going to go directly into your bloodstream, and bypass your gut, which means it will be absorbed way faster. This is what you want when it comes to magnesium supplements. It's not for everyone, but it has worked for me, and may work for you too.

There are many different variations of magnesium oil you can try. You can buy it straight from a health food store, but I'm warning you, you're going to pay a hefty price. You can also buy it straight from Dr. Carolyn Dean's website.

You can also make it yourself.

There is a recipe available in the MAG group, and I'll let you go there to look it up. It's called MAG-A-HOL, simply because it's alcohol and magnesium flakes melted into one. It's supposed to be one of the best types of magnesium oil you could ever make. I highly recommend checking the recipe out.

As for me and my stubbornness, I wanted to come up with my own recipe. I didn't want to put alcohol on my skin everyday, so I developed a recipe with just water. I guess you can't really call it a recipe, because it's so easy peasy simple, but it's the way I do it.

Basically, all I do is buy a bag of magnesium flakes at the health food store. Magnesium flakes are pure magnesium chloride. Normally you just put them in the bathwater and let them absorb. They are quite strong compared to Epson salt, which is a sulfate. We will cover that later.

When I make a batch of magnesium oil, I empty the entire 3.6 kg bag into a 4-liter ice cream pail. I boil regular tap water, and fill up the ice cream pail. I watch the magnesium flakes melt, and then I let it cool. That's it. I'm sure others will say that's not as good, but for me, it's always done the trick.

I put the cooled magnesium oil into plastic containers, and I use a little spray bottle to apply it. But here is where it gets tricky. You can't just immediately douse yourself with it from head to toe. You have to start with one tiny little spray on your skin and see how it will react. This is very important, and I will tell you why.

Your body wants to fight it. Anything good that you introduce into your body, can cause a herxheimer reaction. If you don't know what that is, I would suggest googling it. I could go on and on about it, but basically it is a fighting reaction to good things.

One can develop flulike symptoms, or nasal congestion, or skin rashes, during a herxheimer reaction. You might think that this natural remedy you're taking, is causing you to be sick, but I'm telling you it may not be what it seems. It may be that the natural remedy you are taking, is helping your body so much, and causing a temporary reaction in your body, until you get used to it.

This happened to me with magnesium oil.

I'm here to tell you, proven fact, that I experienced a terrible herxheimer reaction to magnesium oil. My entire body became covered in spots. I looked like I had a case of the measles. Seriously!

I used too much too soon!

As you've probably already guessed, I'm stubborn. I'm hotheaded and extreme. I come by it naturally because I'm a redhead. Funny as it may seem, I really believe it's true. Though I have blonde hair now, my roots are red. A combination of too many highlights over the years, and fading red hair with age. People can't even tell that I once had a head full of red hair. So, with that said, I hope you understand that my stubbornness has been my folly, many a time.

Naturally, I thought spraying almost the whole bottle all over my skin would be so amazing. Well it wasn't. Not only did I get spots over my entire body for a week, I also felt so unwell. I developed a stuffy weird cold, that wasn't like any cold I'd ever had. It almost felt like a fake cold. Looking back, I realize it was a herxheimer reaction, but I didn't really know anything about it at the time.

I also became very lightheaded. The old dizziness reared its ugly head for a short time, but never became a full-blown thing. It's hard to describe, but I knew it wasn't the real dizziness coming back. To this day, I try very hard not to overspray, but if I do and I feel a little lightheaded, I immediately stop. I know the signs of herxheimer now, and I highly respect it. You must respect it also.

The average person would say to just stop what you're doing if you experience the herxheimer reaction. Yes, I would say stop for a time, but don't give it up altogether. Just the simple fact that you are experiencing a herxheimer reaction, tells you that it is good for you, and your body needs to go through that, to reach the next level of health. It's so true. I would highly recommend doing more research on the herxheimer reaction, to fully understand what I'm talking about. Herxheimer reactions are real, and can make your life miserable if you don't understand and respect it.

Today, I use magnesium oil with caution. I spray a maximum of 10 sprays on my skin a day. I know I can slowly build up to more if I want to, but for now, I'm at 10. Ultimately the more magnesium you can get in your system, the better. And no, from what I have found out, you cannot overdose on magnesium. It is impossible. Since the entire body runs on magnesium, there is no real risk other than herxheimer reactions. If you have more magnesium than you need in your system, you'll just pee it out.

My doctor was concerned when I told her how much magnesium I take. She immediately sent me for a blood test to find out if my kidneys were okay. I passed with flying colors. No risk at all. It's something doctors don't seem to understand.

Epson Salt

Epson salt is pure magnesium. It's a sulfate, and therefore cannot be ingested. You can use it in the bath to relax, and you probably never even knew what was in it. Well my friends, it's magnesium.

When I found out that Epson salt was magnesium, I was thrilled. I couldn't believe that I had found a source of magnesium that was cheap and relaxing. All I had to do was dump a couple cups of Epson salt in my warm bath, and let my skin soak it all up. No matter how much Epson salt I put in the bath, or how many times I used it, I never noticed an adverse effect. I haven't experienced one herxheimer reaction with Epsom salt. If you do nothing else in the way of magnesium supplements, do Epson salt baths. You will be pleasantly surprised with the outcome.

Natural calm

This is a powder you put in your drink. I bought a couple bottles of it, and drank it at work. It really helped me calm down, but I found it to be weaker than other supplements. I guess perhaps you could just use more of it, but it's pretty expensive.

I was surprised to find out that it was magnesium citrate. I kind of wanted to limit how much citrate I took in, because of its laxative effect. I assume that's why natural calm seems to be weaker. They don't want everyone running to the bathroom.

If you're interested in this type of supplement, you can find it at your health food store, or in grocery stores and pharmacies. Just be prepared to pay a little more out of your pocket.

ReMag

This product is strictly available through Dr. Carolyn Dean's website. She developed it, and it is said to have no laxative effect. It's available in liquid form. I would recommend checking this out on her website. She has many other magnesium products for sale as well.

Liquid Ionic Magnesium

You drink this. I tried a few bottles of it but I never did really see much of a benefit from it. That's just me though. My personal opinion is that it's a waste of money, because I quickly breezed through a bottle and didn't feel any different. I took about a couple teaspoons of it in the morning, and then a couple in the evening. That quickly depleted my source, that cost me over 30 bucks a bottle.

It only has 25 mg of magnesium per serving, but it is said to be absorbed in the mouth and stomach, rather than digestive system. I guess the idea is that you don't need as much magnesium this way, but I never fully understood this. As I said, I'm not a doctor, and I don't understand all the medical things pertaining to it. I'm just like you, fumbling along trying to make sense of all this information. I have some experience taking this type of magnesium, and just wanted to share that with you.

If you're interested in liquid ionic magnesium, I'd recommend at least trying it. You may find that this type of magnesium works best for you. As I said before, everyone is different, and what works for someone else, may not work for you. It's all about trial and error in finding what suits you best.

Magnesium Bisglycinate

My new best friend. I soon discovered that there is a magnesium supplement out there in pill form, that is not a laxative. Ladies, I give you Bisglycinate. It is a chelate, and is in my opinion the best form of magnesium supplement that you can take. The reason behind this is because it is the most bioavailable. Bioavailable is a fancy word for absorption, so in other words this one is absorbed better in our body.

I have also been told that Magnesium Bisglycinate, somehow bypasses the digestive system and goes directly to the brain. There was a lot of scientific mumbo-jumbo that I discovered about this form of magnesium, but to sum it up it gets absorbed into our blood easier than the rest. You see, magnesium has to be bonded with something in order for us to use it as a supplement. If our bodies can't break that bond to absorb it, we might as well be taking nothing at all, because it won't absorb. That's why Magnesium Bisglycinate is considered to be the best form of magnesium supplement, because it is the most bioavailable.

I know, a lot to take in. It's not exactly easy science for the average brain. It took me years to research all this, and understand enough to even talk about it. Let's face it, the average layperson finds this information difficult. That's why I wanted to write a book about it, to simplify all of the natural remedies for menopause, in a way that we can understand.

Foods with Magnesium

I wanted to lightly touch on foods that contain magnesium, just to let you know that you don't have to spend an arm and a leg on supplements, if you don't want to. I do however believe that the foods that are grown these days, do not contain as much magnesium as they used to. Our soil has been robbed of it over the years, so much so that the mineral is almost depleted.

There are however, some food sources that are still high enough to be beneficial as a good source of magnesium. The shortlist is as follows:

- Dark leafy greens
- Nuts and seeds
- Fish
- Basil lentils

- Whole grains
- Avocados
- Berries
- Bananas
- Dried fruit
- Dark chocolate

These are the highest food sources with magnesium, but there are many other foods that I could list as well. I just wanted to do the top 10.

Calcium

Everyone thinks you're supposed to take magnesium with calcium. But I'm here to tell you, that that was not the case for me. My body had an overabundance of calcium already. The doctor told me to take calcium supplements years ago, and so that's what I did. The result was calcium buildup in my body, so much so, that it was turning me into cement, and making my magnesium deficiency even worse.

You see, magnesium and calcium do work hand-in-hand, but if one outweighs the other, you can run into a lot of trouble. I think calcium supplements do more harm than good. There are so many food sources that we can get calcium from naturally, that we don't have to supplement. But for magnesium, it's hard to get enough from just food.

If you want to take calcium, it's up to you, but I wanted to share my experience with you, so that you could make a proper decision. Because I had a lot of muscle pain prior to taking magnesium, and dizziness also, which indicated magnesium deficiency, I look back now and realize, it was because I was too high in calcium, and too low in magnesium. I was not in balance.

An indication of this was revealed in my saliva. As far back as I can remember, every time I went to the dentist, they would have to chisel away at my teeth, because I had such a huge mineral deposit inside my lower bottom teeth. I remember I would always be so embarrassed, because they kept telling me to brush and floss more. Well, I did, and it never helped.

Prior to my magnesium discovery, I went to the dentist for cleaning. Once again as usual, even going every six months for cleaning, I had a pile of mineral buildup that needed to be chiseled away. Indeed, it was humiliating.

After that last cleaning, I started taking my magnesium, and checking every so often for the usual mineral buildup. It never returned. It was unbelievable. The moment I started taking magnesium, the calcium buildup, which I truly believe it was caused from, had all but disappeared.

Going back to my hygienist for my next cleaning, was a joy. She couldn't believe the mineral deposits were gone. I giggled with enthusiasm as I told her it was because of the magnesium I was taking, and she was very surprised. I'm not sure if she really believed me, but it's true. I also stopped taking calcium as well, but I know it wasn't that alone, because I had the mineral buildup even as a child, and I wasn't taking calcium supplements then. So, for me, I know that it was the lack of magnesium, and then adding it to my diet, that brought balance to my system.

If calcium can do that to my teeth, what has it been doing to the rest of my body? Seriously, I truly believe that taking calcium supplements is a big no-no during menopause. Do we want to become cement? I don't! I refuse to take the junk, and yes, I call it junk. I believe our bodies need magnesium for our bones, more than we need calcium. I believe calcium solidifies cysts in our body, and can cause cancer. But that's just me.

Pink Himalayan Salt

This miracle salt is completely natural, and one of the best salts you can ever ingest. Now, most people believe that you shouldn't have much salt, but I believe otherwise. From the research I've done, I have found that salt is very beneficial. In the old days, they used to consume way more salt and had a lot less diseases.

From the menopausal perspective, the amount of benefit that you get from taking salt every day, is huge. Pink Himalayan salt is packed with minerals. Some of these minerals are magnesium, potassium, iodine, zinc, iron, and the list goes on.

Zinc helps with faster wound healing, and iron helps with formation of hemoglobin in our body, as well as prevents anemia. Together, all the minerals help to maintain a wellness we need during this crucial transition in our lives.

You can replace table salt, with this lovely pink salt as well. In fact, if you find yourself waking up with puffy eyes every morning, it is about time to make the switch. You see, pink Himalayan salt has less sodium than table salt, and it reacts differently in our bodies. It doesn't harm us like table salt does. In fact, it is better for those who suffer from high blood pressure, because it regulates the amount of sodium in our body. With this salt, you have lesser fluid buildup, and lesser swelling of the feet as well.

This lovely pink salt can also flush out toxins, balance your pH level in your body, and enhance blood circulation. It can also enhance your libido. It can reduce muscle spasms and maintain proper electrolyte levels. It can also strengthen your bones because of all the wonderful natural minerals found in it.

I use this salt for everything now. I cook with it. I supplement with it. I ingest it daily, and it has helped me so much. If you would like to do more studies on this type of salt to be sure it's right for you, I would highly recommend finding out as much as you can about it. It really is a wonder salt.

Chapter 2 – Herbs

Vitex

One of the first herbs that I ever started taking was called Vitex. I still take it. It's been a God send to me. In fact, when I run out, I severely miss it. It helps with my hot flashes, and when I forget it, or run out of it, I sweat with a vengeance. I didn't really realize how important it was until the whole city ran out. Yes, indeed, I tried to buy it several different times, but our local health food store kept running out. I told myself it wasn't really that important, so I would wait. My one-week wait turned into two weeks, then three, until an entire month had gone by where I hadn't taken my vitex. Each night I watched my hot flashes intensify, and at first didn't connect the dots. Finally, I thought perhaps it was because of the Vitex. The next day, I got desperate and found a different brand at the grocery store, and decided to try it. I'm glad I did, because almost immediately, my hot flashes became less intense.

What is Vitex you ask? Simply put, it is a berry. Chaste berry to be exact. It's sometimes known as Vitex angus-castus. It can be used as a natural treatment for perimenopause, menopause, and PMS. Most people know this herb as a help for menstruation problems like PMS, but it has also been found to be helpful if you are trying to conceive. There have been numerous reports of women getting pregnant because of Vitex. It has also been reported that Vitex is way more superior than Prozac for treating PMS.

For menopause symptoms, Vitex decreases hot flashes after only eight weeks of use, according to a recent study. But as I said, I can attest to it working way sooner than eight weeks. It also helps decrease night sweats, insomnia, headaches, depression, anxiety, and cravings. It really is a wonder herb.

Vitex is said to balance the hormones. I really found it effective for breast pain and tenderness during perimenopause. In fact, it took it away almost immediately. It makes sense, because this berry is a natural hormone balancer, and has been used for centuries in Asian countries. It also helps with skin issues caused from hormone imbalances. I know people who have used this herb to clear up their severe acne.

The pills are merely capsules of ground-up chaste tree berry. They look gray-green in color, and I usually take two pills in the morning, and two in the evening. It depends on the brand and dosage, but basically, it's recommended that women take anywhere from 500 to 800 mg per day.

St. Johns Wort

I must admit I have never tried this herb. It's always scared me. I know that's silly, but the word reminds me of a witch's brew. I guess it's the word that makes me paranoid. Silly, I know. I've always wanted to find out more about this herb and I'm sure many of you do as well. So here's your chance.

It's often used in combination with chaste tree berry (Vitex). According to a few studies that have been done, the two herbs in combination, can reduce PMS like symptoms in late peri menopausal women, after only 16 weeks. The herb significantly reduced PMS in these study subjects, including bloating, depression, and anxiety. In other studies, specifically targeting postmenopausal women, St. John's Wort reduced hot flashes and depression.

So what exactly is St. John's Wort? Basically it's a beautiful yellow flower from the Hypericaceae family. Its scientific name is Hypericum Perforatum or Hypericum. Not that we need to know that, but it's helpful in understanding what you're putting into your body. Always research before you swallow something.

I was surprised in finding out that this is just a flower. Often I don't take things because I've never heard of them. Even though I research quite a bit, I admit this one stumped me. There are so many natural things that are helpful to us, if we only give it a try. How more natural can something be, than a flower. The only problem I have with some herbs, is the folklore that goes with it. All I really want to know is will it help me? I'm sure that's everyone's question.

I found a lot of research pertaining to this herb, but most of it was wild folklore, and I didn't want to bore you with all the details. I wouldn't have included it in this book if it was only a flower known for its mystical magical folklore. I included it as a remedy, because of studies I had found showing its positive influence on our bodies during perimenopause and menopause.

I hope that you will try this herb, because it has been used safely for over 2000 years. I may even try it myself.

Maca Root

I've never heard of Maca Root, but I was intrigued to learn about it. It's a little root that looks like garlic. It's native to Peru.

How can it help you? It decreases cortisol levels in your body. That's a good thing, because cortisol is a stress hormone, and it regulates how we handle stress in our bodies. Excess cortisol is responsible for osteoporosis, impaired immunity, increased abdominal fat, and reduced muscle mass. If we don't keep our cortisol levels in check during menopause, we will feel very unwell.

Now, I'm not a healthcare professional by any means, and I don't pretend to be one. I'm just a woman who has experimented with a lot of different natural medicines pertaining to menopause, and I want to pass that information along to others. I don't know everything about the human body or how cortisol works exactly, but like everyone of you out there, I try to find out what I can.

Take this information and study it for yourself. I encourage you to become empowered with information. Learn these things and you will discover that you have more control over menopause than you thought you did.

It's recommended that a woman should take anywhere from 1000-2000 mg a day. Because it decreases cortisol levels, it can reduce the effects of stress during this very crazy time in our lives. It is said to lower hot flashes, restlessness, weight gain, fatigue, and improve our libido. And we can all use that!

Black Cohosh

This herb is another wildflower. It's grown naturally anywhere from southern Ontario, to Central Georgia. It's also found as you go West, to Missouri, and Arkansas.

Black Cohosh is said to help prevent hot flashes and night sweats. There's been a lot of research done on this herb, proving that it helps with many other menopausal symptoms as well, including fibroids, hormone imbalances related to diabetes, and improves sleep disruptions.

The recommended dosage is about 80 mg once or twice daily. But like anything, I'd experiment with how you feel when you take it, and see if it is right for you.

Ginseng

I think everyone has heard about this herb. It's well known, but even I didn't know how it could help me during menopause. I was surprised to learn that this fleshy root-looking perennial, was responsible for relieving hot flashes. It is also helpful with vaginal dryness, another frustrating aspect of menopause. I will go over some natural remedies that I personally have found to relieve this lovely problem, later in the book.

Ginseng is also said to improve sexual arousal and increase energy. It can decrease fatigue and depression, and can improve memory and thinking skills.

Recommended dosage is about 600 - 1200 milligrams daily, but it can vary from person to person. You really have to be cautious when trying any natural remedy. I can't stress this enough. No one is the same, and we all react differently to things. What works well with one person may have the adverse effect on another.

There are many alarming side effects to any natural remedy, but I chose not to list them in this book. I wanted to empower women, not defeat them. We have enough things going on inside our menopause brains, that we don't need to worry about every little thing. If we let ourselves be consumed by worry and panic, over all the different side effects attributed to natural medicine, we'll worry ourselves sick.

I encourage each one of you to do your own research on the side effects, because they are not created equal.

Red clover

This is an interesting one. I've never heard of it before. Apparently it's not really red at all, it's hot pink. Here's another example of a beautiful flower that we can eat. It's native to Western Asia, Europe, and Northwest Africa.

How can this help you during menopause? This herb is said to prevent bone density loss. That is invaluable as we age. As I entered menopause, that was one of the major issues I worried about. I wondered if my bones were going to become so fragile that I would break a hip. I've always heard about the elderly falling and breaking a hip, so I thought I had that to look forward to with good old menopause. Just knowing that there are natural things that you can take to prevent loss of bone density, is empowering to me.

Red clover is also said to contain isoflavones. Isoflavones are polyphenolic compounds, also classified as phytoestrogens. Can you guess what these are? Natural estrogen, or should I say compounds with estrogen-like qualities. Now that's amazing! Who would've thought that we could find natural estrogen in nature? Haven't we all thought that the only way to replenish estrogen is synthetically? Not true.

And did you know that soybean and legumes are the riches source of isoflavones? I bet you're going to look at those foods differently from now on. I know *I* will.

So, my dear friends, Red clover is something that I may try, if only for the mere fact that it is an isoflavone, that produces estrogen like qualities naturally.

Evening Primrose Oil

Another pretty yellow flower, this herb can be put directly into your food and used as a good source of essential fatty acids. I didn't know this. In fact, I didn't know much about Evening Primrose Oil. I had heard about it a few years ago, when one of my friends was taking it for menopause, but I didn't know how it helped her.

Evening Primrose Oil is somewhat like Vitex for its healing qualities. It's used for PMS, and balances the hormones. It can be helpful with endometriosis, as well as breast tenderness and hot flashes, during perimenopause and menopause. Usually when I mentioned the word menopause, I clump it all together with peri/pre/post, so I hope you won't be confused as to whether or not this information pertains to you.

Because this herb is botanical, it is often used in soaps and cosmetics. So the next time you see something with this ingredient, you might want to buy it. Not only will it smell nice, but it will be beneficial to you as well.

Dosage varies, so be careful while you experiment with this, and consult a doctor, or naturopath, who can help determine what is right for you.

Red raspberry leaves

Raspberry leaves contain vitamin C. During menopause, vitamin C is essential to our health because it prevents bone density loss, and can actively stimulate bone growth and protect your skeleton. Now that's something.

Not only are red raspberry leaves good for us because of the vitamin C, but it also helps prevent hot flashes. Used in tea, it's an age old remedy for female problems, because it regulates hormones. I wish I would've known this when I was pregnant with my three kids, because this herb also prevents morning sickness. How lovely is that.

Red raspberry leaves also prevent anxiety. It can reduce stress and relax your muscles, because it's infused with B vitamins.

I'm not sure if it will help you, because everyone's different, but it's worth a try. I know that I'm going to be looking for red raspberry tea in the grocery store, the next time I go shopping. I'll be putting my feet up, relaxing with a nice cup of this lovely tea, for sure.

Licorice Root

A study done at Shahid Beheshti Medical University in 2010, has proven that licorice root is effective in reducing hot flashes, adrenal fatigue, mood swings, and depression. This is wonderful news, but for me I want to know why? What is an licorice root, and how does it work to reduce hot flashes?

Firstly, licorice root is a perennial plant that looks like tree branches. Almost like cinnamon sticks. It's often ground-up and put into capsules, but you can even make your own home remedies by adding this root to a tonic or a tea, or in food. It is said to contain stress relieving qualities, because it works on the neurotransmitter, serotonin. It's often used together with ginseng.

This is another herb that contains flavonoids, so it has estrogen-like qualities. It is also dubbed to boost the immune system and prevent heart disease. It is an anti-allergic, anti-inflammatory, anti-arthritic estrogenic. An all around yummy treat.

The next time you have a sweet tooth, grab some licorice and munch away. Not only will it alleviate your cravings, but it will calm you down and relieve your menopausal symptoms as well.

My mouth is watering just thinking about it.

Sarsaparilla

Otherwise known as Smilax Ornate, it is an herb found in Mexico, the Caribbean, and Central America. It's a trailing vine with a prickly stem, used to make a soft drink. Yes, a soft drink. This drink used to be made in the 19th century in the old West. It was quite popular. It tasted like beer, and was often referred to as a 'sissy drink' when ordered at a saloon. Cowboys would drink it before visiting a brothel, because it was said to prevent syphilis and gonorrhea. In fact, from 1820 – 1910, sarsaparilla was registered in the US Pharmacopeia as a valid syphilis treatment.

Nowadays, extensive research has been done on this herb. Along with the healing qualities, it is said to alleviate a great deal of menopausal symptoms. It is said to increase estrogen and progesterone, alleviate joint problems, urinary problems, skin problems, fatigue, and increase your libido.

The herb is believed to have qualities that can flush out toxins, due to its anti-oxidant properties. It's believed to enhance vision as well as nourished the colon and liver. In some cultures, it is used to treat leprosy because of its anti-inflammatory properties. Rheumatism, gout, and arthritis are known to benefit from this herb as well.

There is no doubt in my mind that Sarsaparilla could quite possibly be one of the best 'undiscovered' natural treatments for menopausal symptoms, and old age in general.

I really want to try this, and will be looking for this lovely herb in my local health food store, the next time I'm there.

Holy Basil

Holy Basil is from the mint family. It is an Ayurveda herb as well as an adaptogen. As we have learned already, adaptogen herbs bring you into balance by working with the endocrine system. A.k.a. your hormones.

This herb will calm your system down, and works well with those that are under stress, and in adrenal fatigue. When were stressed, we produce more cortisol, and even when we drink stimulants like coffee or eat a lot of junk food with sugar in it, our cortisol rises. So, when this happens it affects your hormones in a huge way. Holy Basil, because of it's ability to balance hormones, is a great super herb for this issue in particular.

You can use Holy Basil in your cooking, as well as in a tea. I'm excited to purchase this herb and make a tea. I might even grow it in my garden next year.

In conclusion to this chapter, there are many other herbs that may very well be good for menopause, that I haven't covered in this chapter. I didn't include some herbs because there wasn't enough scientific evidence that they were beneficial, but you may find something not on this list that works wonderful for you. If so, I'd love to hear from you.

Chapter 3 - Vitamins

B vitamins

B vitamins should be taken together with magnesium for optimum health during menopause. They include folic acid, thiamin, riboflavin, niacin, pantothenic acid, and pyridoxine. Better known as B1, B2, B3, B5, B6, and B-12.

B vitamins are responsible for a healthy nervous system, a healthy liver, a healthy adrenal gland, sex hormones, and balanced serotonin and neurotransmitters. They all have to do with stress, and during menopause stress can come into play in a big way.

Without B supplements during menopause, we are five times more likely to experience hot flashes. According to one study, low B vitamins attributed to higher stress levels and anxiety in menopausal women.

I find that if I don't take my B-12 and my B-100 supplements everyday, I become a basket case. My stress level soars, and I'm tired all the time. I even found once I started taking B-12, that I didn't need sunglasses so much. I would squint in the sun all the time and could barely handle the brightness. With B-12, my eyesight seems to have improved a great deal.

If you're interested in supplementing with B vitamins, you can get them almost anywhere. I was sucked into thinking the best place to get B-12, was in a health food store. I've purchased it in other places, and I have to say that the health food store is just a money grab. There's nothing wrong with getting B-12 from your local grocery store, even the sublingual kind. They all work fine.

B-12 is not easily absorbed in the body, so the best way to absorb it is sublingual under the tongue. This kind is very expensive at health food stores, but I found another one at my local grocery store that does the same thing. You don't necessarily have to put it under the tongue, you just suck on it like candy, and it slowly absorbs inside your mouth, and that's all you need. Sublingual.

Vitamin C

Vitamin C is a game changer for menopause, because simply put, it can combat vaginal dryness which is the dark side of menopause, and rarely talked about. In our youth we were well lubricated, but menopause changes all that. Not only does our skin get dry, our private parts do as well, and that can become uncomfortable very quickly if we don't do something about it.

Vitamin C will keep us moist. The more you can get, the better. The best sources of vitamin C are natural, so chow down on the oranges. I'd stay away from the vitamin C supplements, and get this lovely vitamin through food.

The following are the top 10 highest foods with vitamin C:

- Citrus fruit
- Yellow bell peppers
- Broccoli
- Kiwi fruit
- Berries
- Tomatoes
- Peas
- Papayas
- Dark green leafy vegetables
- Guavas

Oh, and by the way, studies show that vitamin C can ward off hot flashes as well, so load up with this lovely vitamin as soon as you can.

Vitamin E

Why is vitamin E essential in menopause? Simply put, because research has shown us that vitamin E relieves stress, and stress is a major factor during menopause. Vitamin E is also thought to be an antioxidant, and therefore able to reduce the risk of heart disease.

Supplementing with vitamin E is beneficial during menopause, but there are many great foods that contain natural vitamin E that are much better for you, in my opinion. The top 10 are as follows:

- Nuts
- Sunflower seeds
- Spinach
- Broccoli
- Kiwi
- Mango
- Tomato
- Shellfish
- Fish
- Avocados

Omega-3

Two new studies in Canada, show that omega-3 fatty acids in fish oils, significantly reduces hot flashes and depression.

This one is self explanatory, and I simply wanted to create a list of great omega-3 sources for the menopausal woman. The top 10 are:

- Flaxseed
- Chia seed
- Walnuts
- Caviar
- Oysters
- Soybeans
- Spinach
- Sardines
- Krill oil
- Cod liver oil

Vitamin D

I would completely stay away from vitamin D supplements. Morley Robbins talks a lot about it in the MAG group. I won't go into all the details, because you can look them up yourself, but I *did* want to mention it here.

Vitamin D is a synthetic hormone, that can severely harm us. Anything synthetic can react poorly in our bodies. The best source of vitamin D is from the sun, but if you must take a supplement, go for cod liver oil, or a food source like sardines.

As for redheads, we generate our own vitamin D. I bet you didn't know that. It's truly amazing, but a topic for another discussion.

There are plenty of other good vitamins that I have not listed in this chapter, that may be beneficial as well, but these are the main ones. I hope that you have found this guide helpful, and will follow me along to the next chapter where I get into more non-traditional natural remedies for menopause.

Chapter 4 – Non-conventional Remedies

Turmeric

Golden in color, this lovely perennial plant is from the ginger family, and it really belonged in chapter 2 with the herbs, but I just couldn't put it there. To me it's more than an herb, it's one of the best non-conventional natural remedies in the world. It deserves a class of its own. I've never experienced such a wonder herb as this one.

What they do is grind up this orange root into a powder, and sell it in pill form or powder form. By itself it's not really absorbable, but if you make it into a paste, with pepper, hot boiling water, and an omega-3 fatty acid, you get what we call, Golden Paste.

I make it all the time.

It really is that simple. Boiling water, turmeric powder, oil, and pepper. Mix it up into a paste, let it cool, and put it in the fridge. It keeps for about two weeks. I take about 1 tablespoon in the morning, and 1 tablespoon at night. I built my dosage up very slowly to get my body used to it. That is important, otherwise it will run right through you. This remedy will also cause a Herxheimer reaction, so be careful. Use a little at a time.

So, what are the benefits during menopause? That is the question.

I belong to a Facebook group for turmeric. I actually belonged to two. One of them was started by a veterinarian, who discovered feeding turmeric to animals was hugely beneficial, and prolonged their lives in some instances, and even cured cancer in some animals. I thought, how wonderful. If there had been that much success in animals, how much more so with human beings.

Turmeric is said to be an antioxidant, antimicrobial, anti-cancer, and anti-inflammatory. Curcumin is actually the main ingredient in turmeric, and gives it its bright yellow orange color. Many ethnic groups use it as a spice, but it's healing qualities and therapeutic properties make it much more.

Really, turmeric is relevant to everyone, not just menopausal women. But because it is so beneficial, many of the health disorders that it helps, are in direct relation to menopause.

This lovely spice/herb is one of those super herbs that mimics estrogen in the body. It's called Phytoestrogen. In fact, did you know that Phytoestrogens are often given as alternatives to hormone replacement therapy? Oh yes, there are many studies already done to prove this fact.

It is estrogen deficiency during menopause that causes the hot flashes, mood swings, anxiety, sleeping disorders, vaginal dryness, joint pain, heart disease, and the list goes on. Balancing estrogen levels is key. If we can do that with turmeric, a natural hormone replacement therapy so to speak, we can avoid the dangerous side effects of the drugs prescribed for menopause today.

Turmeric is also a great painkiller. It has analgesic properties, and I can attest to that. It far outweighs acetaminophen and ibuprofen. Studies show that turmeric can help treat muscle soreness caused by menopause, joint pain, and even migraines. Now, ain't that something. And it's not just made up facts. I am living breathing proof of it. Whenever I have any kind of ache or pain, I always take a spoonful of my Golden Paste, and I'm as good as new!

This lovely golden herb has also been proven to be very effective as an antidepressant. Because of the low estrogen in our bodies, we sometimes struggle with depression during menopause, that directly affects our sleep, our stress levels, and even our hot flashes. I have noticed my mood has evened out whenever I take turmeric.

Because turmeric is an antimicrobial, it acts like an antibiotic. Isn't that amazing? So it can fight drug-resistant bacterial infections without the side effects of conventional antibiotics. For most postmenopausal women, this is huge, because as our estrogen levels take a nosedive, vaginal atrophy can sometimes increase, leaving us prone to a gamut of vaginal infections. This is where the anti-bacterial, anti-fungal, and anti-inflammatory properties are put to use.

Yes, you can even use turmeric as a topical treatment.

Some of us struggle with diabetes, autoimmune diseases, and heart disease, even before we reach menopause. As we enter into the change, that all just gets worse. But there is hope. There is hope with turmeric. It can boost our impaired immune systems, and literally heal us from the inside out.

Ethnic families are said to feed their children turmeric milk, especially when they have a fever. It's because it boosts the immune system. Turmeric milk is just a mixture of milk and turmeric. It's not complicated, and easy to make.

Interestingly enough, turmeric can also help you lose weight, and can make you look younger and feel younger. I can attest to that. I feel healthy and young again when I take turmeric.

It's also known to reduce the risk of breast cancer, help preserve bone health, prove therapeutic for arthritis, and be good for heart health. It's a wonder herb if I ever did see one. I will never stop using turmeric, even though my husband gets quite annoyed when he finds yellow stains on the counter. I try not to leave stains when I make my Golden Paste, but sometimes it's unavoidable.

You should know that if you choose to try turmeric as a supplement, you will find stains everywhere except your teeth. Yes, that's right. The yellow won't stain your teeth at all, in fact, turmeric can be used as a teeth whitener. Unbelievable!

You will not be disappointed if you try this lovely herb. There is a special place in my heart for this lovely perennial, that has changed my life so completely. It has brought me back from the brink.

Try it!

Coconut oil

One of the very first natural remedies I tried, is coconut oil. It is God's wonder food. I shovel it in by the spoonful, and I don't get fat, or have any negative side effects.

I can't stress enough about the value of eating good fats during menopause. A lot of people think that you need to do low-fat everything, but from the studies I have read, I know that not to be true. We need good fats for not only our hormones, but for heart health as well. Coconut oil is one of them.

Now, I can tell you that I have spent a small fortune on coconut oil over the years, simply because not all coconut oil is created equal. Some are cold pressed, some have been heated up, and some have filler in. You really have to do your research and find out how it's made before you buy it. The best kind is the cold pressed, because the natural qualities are still there. If you heat it up it destroys the natural qualities that make it so good for you.

And what are the natural qualities?

Coconut oil contains fatty acids, more specifically, medium chain triglycerides. Basically, these fatty acids metabolize differently than other fats in our diet. That's a good thing for menopause, because this means that it is immediately converted into energy for us, and doesn't stick to our waistline.

Coconut oil contains lauric acid like breastmilk does, and has the same lovely qualities. It is an antibacterial, an anti-fungal, anti-viral, and protects the immune system. Ladies, we need all the help we can get with this.

Studies prove that coconut oil is a natural treatment for Alzheimer's, high blood pressure, kidney infections. It also protects the liver.

According to one study done in India, it has been proven to be more effective than conventional treatments for arthritis, and the reduction of inflammation.

It is said to prevent cancer, improve memory and brain function, as well as give us more energy and endurance. It can reduce stomach problems like ulcers, and improve digestion. It can reduce symptoms from pancreatitis and gallbladder issues.

The list goes on and on. It can whiten teeth, improve skin issues, prevent osteoarthritis, and this biggie, type II diabetes. Coconut oil is said to balance the insulin levels in the cells. That's huge!

Coconut oil can help you lose weight, and build muscles at the same time you lose fat. Now that's incredible. It's also a proven treatment for yeast infections, and Candida. It has antiaging qualities as well, so for pre/peri/post menopausal women, it's a win-win situation, especially because it balances hormones, and yes, even wards off hot flashes.

I would highly suggest trying coconut oil. I take at least 1 tablespoon a day. I just shovel it in like peanut butter, as crazy as that sounds. I've tried other methods of ingesting it, like mixing it in food or cooking with it, but for me it was just easier to use as a supplement.

I definitely felt a benefit immediately, when I first started using it. I plan to continue supplementing with coconut oil every day. It does not harm me at all, and I've been taking it for over three years. When I first started taking it, everyone gave me grief, saying it was totally unhealthy, because it was fat, and I shouldn't believe everything I read on the Internet. But that wasn't the case at all. Don't listen to the naysayers, try it for yourself. It may very well be, what you need to push you through menopause.

Make sure if you do try it, you look around first, before buying the most expensive. I bought the most expensive, and I didn't see a major difference. It was all in my head. I was fed this mumbo-jumbo from the health food store telling me, I had to spend over 90 bucks to get the right one for the most benefit. In a sense, I was brainwashed into spending 90 bucks for a small tub of coconut oil. That didn't make sense to me over the long term, so I looked into different kinds. As long as it is cold pressed, and organic, it's fine. Really it is. Even if its lightly warmed during processing, it's still good. At least in my opinion it is.

I now buy coconut oil at my local grocery store, and I pay way less. I still feel the same benefit. And here's a little secret, ladies. You can use it as a feminine hygiene product. Yes! What I mean by this is self-explanatory, I hope, but if you need a little bit more detail, here it goes. You can use coconut oil daily, as of vaginal moisturizer and protector from disease, because of its wonderful antibacterial, antifungal, antiviral qualities. This is amazing news for the menopausal woman, because as we age, we become drier where we once were moist, and that makes us susceptible to all kinds of vaginal infections and uncomfortableness.

Using coconut oil as a lube, makes total sense. You can even take a quarter teaspoon of coconut oil, drop it in Saran wrap, wrap it up into individual bullet looking suppositories, and freeze. Once frozen, you can unwrap and insert into the vagina. For those who need this cool lubricated support, I say, go for it girl! Tried, tested, and true!

And for all those women who are wondering if you can use it as a lube for sex, yes you can! You can also use it before and after, as a soap. Yes, a soap! It's the best soap you'll ever use, and best deodorizer as well!

I bet you'll be running to the store for coconut oil now! Wink!

Kombucha Tea

What on earth is Kombucha Tea?

Well, if you haven't heard of it yet, it's the best drink in the world, at least for me anyway. I first heard about it from a friend who invited me over one day, to have a taste and learn how to make it. She also gave me a little starter kit so I could make it myself. To tell you the truth, I was scared to drink it, and never thought I'd be making it myself.

But who knew. It was actually good. I quickly learned that it is a probiotic. It's actually one of the best probiotics we can take. If you don't know what probiotics are, simply put, they are tiny little bugs in our digestive system, that help us have a healthy gut. I know that sounds gross, but it's a layman's term to help you understand. Our bodies are full of bugs, good and bad. Without them, we would die. Sorry to burst your bubble, but that is the truth. It's the way it is, and most people don't even know it.

I was one of them.

My general mentality was, keep myself healthy, eat well, and I won't have any kind of bugs in me. Not true. We need micro organisms in our body to keep us alive, to help us absorb the nutrients in our food, and for good overall health.

One of the reasons why I think my magnesium was low, is because I can't absorb it very well. In fact, prior to taking natural remedies, I had a very poor gut flora. I think it happened right from birth. It's said to be something that gets passed down in utero. As we age and eat poorly, it just gets worse. Some call it a leaky gut, but basically it is an unhealthy digestive system. Probiotics can fix that over time. And it does take time.

I have been working on my gut issues for a long time, trying to help with absorption of vitamins and minerals. I have seen a great improvement since drinking my own Kombucha Tea, but there are many other types of probiotics you can take. Yogurt is a probiotic, but you have to make sure of that. There are many yogurts out there that have pretty poor probiotic levels. Read the label.

I also like to eat sauerkraut, because it is very high in probiotics. Anything fermented is a probiotic: pickles, kefir, dark chocolate, ocean-based plants, raw cheese, soy milk, olives. They are yours to discover.

Probiotic foods and drinks will not only help with your gut absorption, but boost your immune system, prevent bladder infections, heal inflammatory bowel disease, manage eczema, reduce flu and colds, fight foodborne illnesses, lose weight, lower cholesterol, manage autism, treat cancer, treat kidney stones, acne, and even prevent cavities and gum disease. It's incredible!

Surprisingly, it is said that Kombucha tea can be used topically too. Yes! It soothes vaginal atrophy, vaginosis, and even prevents these things. Soak a tampon in Kombucha tea, and insert. The (good) bacteria will bring back normal flora in your vagina. Specifically, lactobacillus, something we lose when we reach menopause. This loss of good bacteria can cause all sorts of problems like atrophy, and yeast infections, and even affect the bladder in a negative way.

I read a new study about the real causes of yeast infections, and bladder infections, and it is said that vaginal flora is responsible. Using yogurt as a cure for yeast infections, has been an age old practice. Why? Because it contains probiotics like Kombucha tea. It contains the good bacteria that is missing.

Now, I wouldn't have told you this little secret if I hadn't tried it myself. I was literally shocked when I tried Kombucha tea topically, when I had some nagging vaginal irritation, pain, itching, and bladder issues. It took it all away. Fast! And not only that, it cures hemorrhoids almost instantly.

I would advise proceeding with caution. Try this at your own risk, as not all women react the same, and this is a very controversial and unproven method. But if you suffer from vaginal atrophy, you will be willing to try almost anything.

So how do you make Kombucha tea?

Firstly, I just want to say that you don't have to make it. You can actually buy it from a health food store like pop. It gets expensive because, for me, I wanted to drink it daily. I didn't want have to buy it every day. As I said before, I'm stubborn.

Remembering back to my friend who gave me a starter kit, as I said before, I was apprehensive about making it. She showed me this big glob of what looked like rotten moldy flesh. Yes, you read that right. It's called a 'mother' or 'scoby' and that's how you start Kombucha Tea.

You might have heard about apple cider vinegar, well that has a 'mother' in it too. It's very similar.

It was hard to get my head around it at first, because the blob, or scoby, looked so gross. Really it's not though, it's actually very clean and it doesn't smell at all. In short, it is what is needed for fermentation to start. And I just wanted to point out that this fermentation process is not alcohol. You are not making wine.

In short, I'll give you the rundown of my process for making Kombucha tea, but if you want to watch a video on how to make it, you can find it on my YouTube channel called *Kat Fit.*

Basically, all I do is boil a pot of water, take it off the stove and cool it, and put 4-6 teabags in it. I just use regular black tea. While it's still hot, I put 2 cups of sugar in it. The little bugs love the sugar and eat it all up, so the finished product is not sweet or bad for you, because there is no trace of sugar once it's fermented.

After the pot of tea is cooled, I put it in two large glass jars, add regular tap water, and put a scoby on top. I cover it with some kind of breathable fabric, and an elastic band to hold it in place over the mouth of the jar. You want the tea to breathe. If you put a lid on it, it will go bad. If you don't put a cover of some sort on it, flies will get in, and it will go bad.

You leave it to ferment for at least two weeks, but I leave mine sometimes for a month or more. When it's ready, I take off the scoby, strain the tea, and put it into bottles or containers, and put it in the fridge to drink.

Just a note about the scoby: When I received the starter kit for my friend, it was just some fermented Kombucha tea in a jar. She told me to leave it on the shelf until it formed a film on top. That film is your new scoby.

But as I said, if you just want to watch the video on how I make Kombucha tea, please go to my YouTube channel.

Just a word of caution, as with anything that is fermented, you need to have a clean kitchen and use clean utensils. If you make this tea, you must know that you are doing this at your own risk. I am not responsible for anyone poisoning themselves. A lot can go wrong when making your own Kombucha Tea, so do the research for yourself before even starting it. If that scares you, then perhaps buying it from the health food store is a better option for you, either that, or choose one of the probiotic foods that I mentioned.

The most important thing is that you get enough probiotics. How you want to do that, whether that be making Kombucha tea, or eating sauerkraut, or yogurt, or buying
probiotic pills, is up to you. The main thing is that you're getting probiotics, the how and the where you get it, is not as important.

Best wishes on your Kombucha tea adventure, if you do try to make it. Let me know how it goes. I'd love to hear from you.

Aroma Therapy

Aroma therapy is something I'm not familiar with, but I will try to give you enough information to form a decision as to whether or not you want to use this as a form of menopause therapy.

The best way to do aromatherapy for menopause, is in the bath. What you would do is you would choose essential oils, and put them in a hot bath, and soak in it. The aroma is said to have properties to help during menopause. I would add Epsom Salt to that lovely warm bath, so you can soak in magnesium at the same time.

Some of the essential oils that are helpful for aromatherapy during menopause are as follows:

- Peppermint - helps with hot flashes, headaches, fatigue, sweating
- Chamomile Roman - helps with skin problems, insomnia, headaches, achiness
- Basil - helps with fatigue, lethargy, lack of concentration
- Geranium - helps with depression, irritability, dry skin, balancing emotions
- Cypress - helps with hot flashes, irritability, fluid retention, sweating
- Clary Sage - helps with disturbed sleep, sweating, hot flashes

Aromatherapy seems to be more basic than I thought, so definitely I will give this a try. I hope you will as well.

Acupuncture

Acupuncture is another area that I have no experience in, but I've heard from many people that it has helped them extremely during menopause.

The Chinese believe that our bodies contain channels of energy like rivers, that nourish your tissues. They believe that these channels of energy can be disrupted when we go through emotional or physical trauma.

In order to re-establish balance in this river of energy, they stick very fine needles in certain points in your body, that are said to regulate the flow of energy and get it back to normal.

Whether you believe in the Chinese explanation of what is happening when the body gets unbalanced or not, is up to you. I personally don't believe it, and you may want to hear the scientific explanation if you're like me. As soon as I heard it, I started thinking a little bit differently about it.

Scientifically speaking, when you stick a needle into your skin, it immediately stimulates the nervous system, which then releases chemicals into your muscles, brain, and spinal cord. We all know that our spinal cords for example, control our entire body with all the nerves that run through it.

Consider when a chiropractor manipulates your spine. Headaches can be taken away, dizziness, aches and pains, even controversial ailments like colic in babies, has been known to be corrected with chiropractic manipulation. All of this has ties to the spinal cord. It makes sense that if you manipulate the spinal cord, muscles, and your brain, by sticking needles in it, something profound will happen. It only makes sense that your body will act differently.

I'm not sure if I will try it, but I am curious about it because of the good things I've heard from menopausal women. I wanted to look up the benefits, so you will be informed as to how this may possibly help you.

Acupuncture is said to relieve hot flashes, stress, and insomnia. It is said to improve your quality of life immensely during menopause, by balancing the hormones. Acupuncture is also said to relieve not just physical symptoms, but mental as well.

This type of therapy is not for everyone, as it involves needles, and needles are something that most people are generally afraid of. The needles are very small, however, but they are still needles. Many have overcome their fear though, and I would encourage you if you're interested in this, to try it, because they say you don't even feel the needles.

So ladies, give it a try, and let me know how it goes.

Molasses

I just wanted to cover briefly on natural Blackstrap molasses. I take a tablespoon every day, and have for a long time. For a while I stopped taking it, but recently started up again. There are so many different natural remedies out there, that if you took everything, it would be exhausting to keep up. You really have to pick and choose your remedies, and develop a plan of action that you can follow on a daily basis. If you have too much on your list it becomes overwhelming.

If molasses is something you want to pursue as a natural remedy, you might be interested to know that it is jam-packed with natural minerals. The only downfall that made me stop taking it for a while, was that it doesn't taste very good. Sure, you can disguise it, and put it into coffee or foods or a warm cup of milk, but I found that I could still taste it. If you can get over the taste, then go for it. The benefits are huge.

One of the best uses for molasses, is as a sleep aide. As we enter menopause, we find it difficult to stay asleep. Not necessarily *fall* asleep, but *stay* asleep. Molasses helps you stay asleep, because it's natures melatonin. It aids in the production of serotonin, melatonin, and dopamine. It works better than any sleeping pill on the market, and is usually used in conjunction with Pink Himalayan salt. But of course, every (body) is different, so proceed with caution.

If you take only 1 tablespoon of blackstrap molasses a day, you will be taking in most of the vitamin B complex except for vitamin B1. It contains 20 percent iron, and happens to be the riches source of natural iron. It also contains 15 percent natural calcium (the kind of calcium you want to take) and 20 percent potassium. It contains natural magnesium, as well as trace amounts of zinc and copper.

Studies have proven that Blackstrap molasses is effective in restoring hair loss and color. It also helps fight dementia, arthritis, dermatitis, fatigue, high blood pressure, magnesium deficiency, nerve problems, and the list goes on. It truly is a magnificent natural vitamin and mineral superfood. I love this black goo. It's liquid gold, black gold. Try it, and you may find its benefits to be invaluable.

Apple Cider Vinegar

Apple cider vinegar is just fermented apple juice. It contains a 'mother' like Kombucha tea, and it is very bitter. I took it every day for a while, until I couldn't stand the bitterness anymore. This is something I overwhelmed myself with, but it doesn't have to be that way for you.

If Apple cider vinegar is something you want to try, I suggest adding it to your diet very slowly. You don't want to be crazy like me, and drink half a cup, or quickly give it up. You can add this to your cooking, and disguise the taste. I should've done that, but I was using it more so as a supplement.

Apple cider vinegar is an natural antioxidant, and has the ability to flush toxins from your body. It also alkalizes the body and will help it alleviate hot flashes, and night sweats. It will even help you sleep. Some women have reported that it has taken their hot flashes away.

Protein Powders

I wanted to emphasize the importance of protein powder during menopause. Strange, I know, but it is way more important than most people realize. Sure, you can eat meat and get your protein that way, but most people don't get enough protein, no matter how much meat they eat. For some crazy reason, society has become scared to death to eat red meat, and good quality protein sources. I can't emphasize enough that the menopausal woman needs that protein more than any age group.

As we go through menopause, if we don't take care of our muscles, we are in big trouble. We need to build muscle mass, because as we age and lose estrogen, that gets distributed differently in our bodies, and that can quickly soar out of control.

Some people say protein powder is not natural, but I'm here to tell you that you can get many different kinds of natural protein powders at the health food store. You can even make it yourself. It can even be completely plant-based if that's what you want.

No matter what source of protein you take, whether that be in the form of a powder, natural, plant-based, vegetable-based, or whatever, the benefits are huge. If you keep your protein intake up daily, you will certainly battle the bulge during menopause.

I take protein powder at least three or four times a week, to make sure I have enough. I've tried all different kinds, and for me personally, it doesn't really matter whether it's made from whey, or peas, or what have you. Just get the protein. You'll be glad you did.

Exercise

This is a no-brainer. We all know that exercise is key during menopause. We don't have to be told to go to the gym, or go for a walk. We just know. It isn't always easy to find time in our busy day to get the exercise we need, so I just wanted to give you a few pointers of what has helped me.

I'll go more into detail in chapter 6, but I just wanted to say that not all exercise is created equal. You don't have to work out like a crazy woman to lose weight and keep yourself fit. In fact, if you go too crazy at the gym, your adrenal system won't like it. If you're already suffering from adrenal fatigue, you will only make it worse if you burn yourself out at the gym.

I want to introduce a different mentality for menopausal women regarding exercise. Rather than plan a workout routine, I have found it better to keep it simple. What I mean by that is, to just do what you enjoy because you enjoy it.

I have done the three days a week at the gym thing, and I can tell you it's not all it's cracked up to be. In fact, it can become quite a bother. I don't say this lightly, because there are many who do this and that's fine, but my experience is different. I just wanted to enlighten you.

After working a busy day at the office, the last thing I want to do is go to the gym after work. It wasn't always like this, but my attitude about it changed after a while. With so many of us being stressed and short for time, I started to question whether going to the gym was the only way I could get proper exercise.

I would run on the treadmill, wear my nice workout clothes and feel good about myself, do a few weights, stretches, and go home. When I got home, I didn't have a lot of time left in my evening. I still had to make supper and get the house work done. That was exhausting. Was it really the only way?

I began regretting the gym. If that's you, you must stop and find another way. If you absolutely adore the gym, keep going. Ladies, it's about happiness, not image. We can get our exercise in other ways.

When I started changing my attitude about exercise, I found I became a healthier woman. I started going for walks simply because I love walking. I began going for bike rides simply because I loved riding my bike. I didn't find it a chore. If it's a chore, it will not benefit your body, because you will be stressed, and the stress will work against you.

I found another way to burn my fat, maintain my muscle mass, keep myself toned, and be happy. It doesn't always have to be the traditional exercise that people think. For example, it can be exercising with a hula hoop. I know someone who does this and she is happy when she works out. It can be yoga. It can be canoeing. It can be speed walking, or a gentle light walk down by the river, smelling the roses and enjoying the warm summer breeze. That's adequate exercise for the body, soul, and mind. Don't be fooled into thinking that the gym is the only way.

I have also developed a life-changing exercise/eating program that we will discuss in chapter 6. It has changed my life and given me back my health.

Ladies, if you exercise to be happy, you will be fit body soul and mind.

Sleep

I wanted to spend a little time talking about sleep. During menopause, as I said before, it's not easy to *stay* asleep. Because of our declining estrogen, our sleep patterns change. We find ourselves waking up in the middle of the night, and not being able to fall back asleep.

Helpful suggestions are making sure your bedroom is completely dark; going to bed at the same time every night; not staying up late; not having a nap in the middle of the day; not looking at the clock every hour. And this one is my favorite: holding your pee as long as you can. I know, probably not the best advice, but it works for me. If I get up in the middle of the night to go to the bathroom, I often can't fall back asleep. If I limit how much water I drink before I go to bed, and hold my pee as long as possible, I sleep better.

Also, installing a good ceiling fan above your bed is a lifesaver. If you can't do that, you need to get an oscillating fan beside your bed. If hubby doesn't like it, too bad. Most of the time they have no idea we struggle with night sweats as much as we do, or hot flashes, that wake us up in the middle of the night. Sometimes, no matter how many supplements we take, we still struggle with some degree of night sweats on and off. When that happens, we have to cool off quickly. That's why you need a fan my friends. I would not be able to survive without one.

Sure, we can take supplements, and try all the different natural remedies I've covered in this book, but our behavior determines our sleep pattern as well. If we follow these simple rules, and get the sleep that we need, menopause is so much easier to get through when were not so tired.

Chapter 5 – Mind Body Therapies

Meditation and Positive Affirmations

One of the best ways to deal with menopause, is to have a positive attitude. I know for myself, if I am continuously negative, my symptoms tend to get worse. That's the case with everything in life, if we have a poor attitude.

If you want to thrive during menopause, you really have to take time out for yourself, and meditate. Now, meditate means something different for everyone. It can be as simple as having some quiet time before your day starts, and thinking about your life, or thinking about nothing at all. It can be a down time for your mind to rest, or it can be an active deliberate thought pattern.

How ever you want to define meditation, my point remains the same. If we don't stop and rest for a few moments throughout the day, depression can easily set in. Life can get so busy sometimes, we wonder why we're even doing what we do. It can become overwhelming depending on our workload, our debt load, our responsibilities, or everything combined. If we let our lives become overwhelming, menopause will become overwhelming.

There are a few different meditation techniques that you can try.

Techniques like hypnosis, and guided imagery, have been helpful to many during menopause. The premise behind it is to calm you naturally, by using music or words to sooth. I have experimented with using words of affirmation, as I struggled with self-image. It worked wonders. I would highly recommend it.

An example of that is with sleeping habits. I was having such a hard time sleeping in general, but more so whenever I went on a trip. Anxiety would build because I knew that I wouldn't get the proper sleep that I needed, to have an enjoyable time. It was quite bothersome to me, because it got to a point where I didn't even want to go anywhere, because I was afraid I wasn't going to get the proper sleep.

Guided imagery helped. I developed a little catchy phrase, and during my walks, I repeated it over and over. It went something like this: "Every time I go on a trip; I sleep like a baby. I mean, every single time without fail." I said this phrase for about two or three weeks, before I went on my trip, and it worked. I was totally shocked.

My brain believed what I told it. Ladies, whatever you feed into your brain, will be what you believe. It's incredible, really. It explains how we can have low self-esteem by believing what we're thinking about ourselves. I encourage you to explore this wonderful technique, because if we speak truth about ourselves, we can change our negative self-image.

As for menopause, if we speak truth about our circumstance, we will believe it. Try making up a song about getting rid of hot flashes. Sing it to yourself every day, and see if it works. I haven't yet tried making up phrases regarding hot flashes yet, but I plan to. I'd love to hear from anyone who has successfully mastered this technique.

Another technique is what I call a cold transfer. Basically, it's pretending to get rid of your hot flash by transferring it somewhere else. You might think this is a bunch of baloney, but I've tried it and it really works.

One day I was sitting in the car waiting for my husband, and the windows were foggy and cold because it was raining out. I started having a hot flash, and thought I'd experiment with this cold transfer idea I had heard about. I put my hot hand on the cold window, and envisioned transferring that hot flash to the window. Well, wouldn't you know it, my hot flash disappeared instantly.

There is one more technique I would like to inform you about, and that is called the tapping technique. I've tried it a few times, but haven't been disciplined about it. The way it works is similar to acupuncture, and is an energy psychology technique. I found it quite interesting.

They call it EFT for short. It stands for Emotional Freedom Technique. In short, you tap certain trigger points in your body, to relieve your symptoms of menopause, and repeat a positive script you make up. For example, "Hot flashes no longer exist in my body."

Popular trigger points are the top of your head, the eyebrow point, side of your eye, under the eye, the rib point, under the arm, under the nose, chin point, the collar point, and many more. It truly is fascinating what the brain will believe if you tell it something.

I won't go into too much detail with the exact process, because it's quite lengthy, but I encourage you to look up a YouTube video on tapping for menopause relief, if you're interested. The best way to learn sometimes is by visually seeing it done. At least that's how I learn.

Motivational speakers

I wanted to include motivational speakers in this book, because they have helped me more than words can say. During menopause, you need all the help you can get, and sometimes, let's face it, our friends aren't always there for us. Some of us don't even have close friends, or don't want to burden them with our problems.

I'm here to tell you there is hope.

Thanks to YouTube, you can look up almost any motivational speaker and be encouraged. I like to listen to Tony Robbins specifically, as well as Brendon Burchard. These two guys, even though they are guys, have really helped encourage me during menopause. Not because they speak about it, but because they're good at what they do. They encourage and motivate.

I think I have listened to almost every single one of Brendon Burchard's videos. When I'm down, its the first one I go to. He talks about self-esteem, and how to handle negative people, and how to change your life for the better.

Don't underestimate what motivational speakers can do for you. There are many female motivational speakers as well. The resources available on YouTube for free are endless. I would highly recommend listening to motivational speakers, if you are struggling with the many changes during menopause.

It isn't always about our physical changes during menopause, it's also mental. Our lives are changing. We're not the young version of ourselves anymore. We have to reinvent ourselves, and that is not easy. Some of us have a difficult circumstances pertaining to health. Some of us have difficult financial circumstances. Some of us have difficulty coping with an empty nest.

It's okay to ask for help. It's okay to seek advice, even if no when else in the world knows or cares. Do it for yourself!

Prayer

I will just come out and say that I'm a religious person. Even if you're not, you can still consider this technique. Prayer. I wanted to briefly cover on this because I feel that it is important to many. If it's not important to you, feel free to skip it.

When I have a bad day and I don't think anyone cares, I know that God does. I believe that Jesus Christ is God, and can save me from not only my sins, but my difficult circumstances. And menopause fits right into that category.

We are prone to depression during menopause, and our lives are so full of change with our unpredictable hormones, that many of us can barely cope some days. I'll be the first one to raise my hand and say that menopause is not easy.

I don't want to pretend that prayer will make it all better, because menopause won't suddenly disappear when we pray, or magically turn us into a 25-year-old. But mentally and emotionally, I have found that prayer gives me the help that I need to persevere through the storm, instead of succumb to its devastation.

Laughter

Ladies, if you can learn to laugh at yourself, you can get through anything. I don't know what it is about laughter, but it puts everything back into perspective. It's like a switch. When you're miserable, and you're wallowing in your own sorrows, you develop a negative brain pattern. Laughter switches your brain back to the positive.

I can't even count how many times I have seen this technique used to change negative circumstances into positive ones. Some people are just better at it than others, and know that adding a little joke into a negative discussion, will get everybody back in a good mood. I don't know if I'm very good at that, but I can certainly laugh at myself.

Being so serious all the time, is not good for us. Find things to laugh about during menopause. Bring your smile back. Look up funny pictures of ladies fanning themselves during a hot flash. Post it on Facebook. Share your own stories.

Make a cognitive effort to laugh every day. It's a choice. I believe laughter is one of the best, if not superior, natural remedies for menopause. Everything changes when we giggle, our brain waves, our chemistry, our demeanor.

Laugh! It will literally change your life!

Chapter 6 -IF

I decided to leave the best for last. Ladies, I introduce you to Intermittent Fasting. Most people have not even heard of such a thing. If they have, their attitude is usually quite negative. People think it's bad for your body. People think that you're going to be starving yourself to death, or that you become anorexic. Generally, they think intermittent fasting is some crazy fad that doesn't work.

I am here to give you living breathing proof, that it does in fact work. It can be the most influential natural menopause remedy that you will ever try.

As I entered into menopause, I began to put on weight. I had never struggled with weight my entire life. I could always eat whatever I wanted without any negative effect.

Menopause changed all that. I grew bigger and bigger by the day, and it seemed like it was spiraling out of control. I had no waist at all, and a big belly. I didn't even recognize myself anymore. I was uncomfortable in my own skin. I had terrible rib pain, and I couldn't figure out why at first. Then, I started realizing it was all the extra fat hanging on my ribs. I couldn't get comfortable.

My work shirts were getting so small that I had to literally stretch them over my growing arms, just to be comfortable. Looking back, I shake my head. I knew I had to do something soon or I was going to suffer the consequences of this extra fat. I knew that if I could see my fat, then there must be fat around all of my major organs as well, and that was not good.

At that time, I was awaiting the birth of my first grandchild. I wanted to be healthy so that I could run around and play with her. I would spend hours crying, because I knew that I couldn't even go for a walk without being tired. How was I going to be the active grandmother that I had always dreamed of?

I tried everything to lose the weight. I tried eating like a bird. I tried eating only vegetables. I tried speed walking. I tried going to the gym. Nothing helped. I was so frustrated that I couldn't lose the weight that I had put on seemingly overnight.

Then one day it all changed. I found something called the 5:2 Fast developed by a doctor in the UK named Michael Moseley. I read his research on this type of fasting, and it was fascinating. Not only did he equate fat loss with this program, but he tried it himself. He was his own guinea pig, and that is what sold me.

I found a Facebook group for the 5:2 Fast, and discovered there were many successful weight loss stories with this program. I was determined to try it myself, even though I didn't tell a soul what I was doing. I didn't want to fail. I thought it probably wouldn't work, so I didn't want to broadcast what I was doing... Unless it actually worked.

Well, it actually worked. I lost a total of 50 pounds in a two-year timeframe. I discovered that you need to lose the weight slowly, because you want it to be maintainable in the long term. It's been three years, and I have managed to sustain it without any effort at all. Intermittent Fasting has become a way of life for me. It's just a new way of eating.

The idea behind intermittent fasting, is the eat-stop-eat method. It's a shock to your system when you don't eat, and it's that shock that signals your body to grab some food now, while it still can, because who knows if it will get anything more. So, what your body does in that circumstance, is it starts burning fat for fuel instead of sugar. Normally our bodies just burn the sugar that we eat, but when we fast, we dip into our reserves so to speak. Basically, it uses up our fat reserves.

You want your body to burn the fat that it's been storing for so long. The way you get it to do that, is to trick it. You've got to freak your body out by making it think it's starving. Really you're not starving. What I quickly learned was that I don't need quite as much food as I thought I did. In fact, menopausal women aren't as active as twentysomethings. If were not as active, we don't need as much food. That's a fact.

I began to realize that I was overeating. Yes, even when I was trying to lose weight, before I tried intermittent fasting by eating like a bird, I was still overeating. I couldn't believe it. This was a hard one to wrap my head around, and if you try intermittent fasting, it will be a hard one for you to wrap your head around too. We simply do not need all that food. We as a society overeat, period!

Who made up the rule that we need three square meals a day anyway? The food and drug administration? Could it be that they want us to over eat so we overspend? Who says we need to snack all the time? Who says we need food every two hours?

I started questioning everything.

As I became more curious, I gained valuable education along the way. One of the things I found out, was something called body mass index (BMI). Basically, this is your body weight in relation to your height. There are many calculators online that will help you determine what your BMI is. This is helpful, because it will show you just how overweight you really are, and what your ideal weight should be. Once you have a starting point, you know what direction you need to go in.

I knew what direction I needed to go in, and I knew it wasn't going to happen overnight. That is probably one of the hardest hurdles to get over when doing intermittent fasting. I know people who have tried it for a short period of time, and said there was no benefit whatsoever. Maybe for some that is the case, but for the average person, all it takes is a little patience and time.

You can also calculate how many calories you need for the week, according to your height, age, and weight. There are many online calculators for this as well, and the reason I bring it up, is because once I realized that it's all about my caloric intake, I had power and knowledge to do something about it. I also learnt that my daily caloric intake, was not as important as my weekly caloric intake. This was a shocker to me, because I had to learn that it wasn't as much *what* you eat, as it is *when* you eat.

I quickly put a couple calorie counter apps on my phone, and started keeping track of how many calories I was actually taking in. This was another shocker. I couldn't believe just one iced lemon drink was over 500 calories. That's crazy. Even one cup of milk is over 100 calories. At first I went around thinking, at this rate, reducing my caloric intake is going to be nearly impossible.

Let me tell you, it is quite the opposite. There are many paths to success with intermittent fasting, and I will briefly go over the ones that I have tried.

Firstly, I just wanted to add that if you currently struggle with any type of eating disorder, or have ever struggled with any type of eating disorder, intermittent fasting is probably not for you. I would seek a doctor's approval before ever attempting this way of eating. It may be, given your history, that intermittent fasting may spiral out of control. I would never want that to happen to you, so please be careful. Do your own research, as I am merely stating what has worked for *me*. If you do try intermittent fasting, it's at your own risk, and I am not responsible for anyone who may try this. That said, I will proceed with the information I gathered over time, from my own experiences.

5:2 Fast

In short, the five and the two represent the days of the week.

We normally eat seven days a week. This type of fast breaks those seven days up. Five of those days are what we call eat days, and two of those days are fast days.

The idea behind this type of fast, is to choose two intermittent days to fast. I chose my fast days to be Mondays and Thursdays. The premise behind this particular fast, is that men are allowed 600 calories, and women are allowed 500 calories on fast days. If you consider that one glass of milk is over 100 calories, then you will understand, that does not allow you much.

When I started the 5:2 Fast, I counted my calories up to 500, and that's what I ate on Monday. It was nothing more than a little bit of salad and a couple glasses of milk. Like I said, not much.

I calculated my calories as I did this week by week, for about a month. I didn't see a change in my weight but I was determined to continue. I decided to stop counting calories and just eat nothing on my fast days. All I had was water, and I started to look forward to my fast days, because I felt this cleaned feeling in my body when I did it.

They say the first two weeks of any fasting program is the hardest, because it takes approximately two weeks for your body to learn to burn fat for fuel instead of sugar. Most of the cravings you experience are because your body is crying for sugar, because we always have given it sugar. Once we get over that, things start changing.

After a couple months of doing the 5:2 Fast, secretly I might add, I started seeing my weight change. I couldn't believe it when I stepped on the scale. I had dropped 10 pounds. That was huge because I had tried everything up to this point, and nothing would budge that number on the scale. I was ecstatic.

People started noticing I looked younger and healthier. Does weight gain make you look older? What I found out from my studies, is that intermittent fasting has a lot more benefits than just weight loss. It brings back that youthful glow.

I follow the 5:2 Fast to this day, and it's been about three years. I love it. I would never go back to the old way of eating. In total, I have lost 50 pounds and feel great. I lost my belly I've had since I gave birth to my three children. I feel youthful and in better shape than I have my entire life. Did you know fasting mimics exercise in the body? Yes!

There are so many benefits to fasting. I need to write a whole book just on that. In fact, I already did, but the day I finished the book, my computer crashed and I lost everything. I was devastated. I still am. Maybe one day I will rewrite that book.

16:8 Fast

Another type of intermittent fasting is called the 16:8. Now, this type of fast is not about the days of the week, but the hours in the day. Sixteen, meaning how many hours you fast, and eight, meaning how many hours you eat. It's actually more simple than it sounds.

You count the hours that you sleep as fasting hours. This type of fast is easier for those who don't want to miss a whole day of eating. You eat supper, and don't have any snacks after 8 PM. If you wake up at 8 AM for example, you've already fasted for 12 hours. By noon you can start eating again. That's sixteen hours of fasting, and you'll have an eight-hour window in which to eat. Simple, isn't it?

I do this type of fast as well, just to give my body a little bit of a shocker. You see, our bodies are creatures of habit, so if we do one thing for a length of time, it starts to become wise to it, and doesn't respond as easily. We've got to switch things up every now and then, so I alternate between the 5:2 and the 16:8.

There is also the 4:3 Fast, which is self-explanatory: Four eat days, three fasts days. Basically, you have to find a method that is right for you when it comes to intermittent fasting. Many claim their way to be the best way, but really every body is different and responds differently, so you have to experiment.

Long Fasts

I wouldn't rule out long fasts. At first I did, because I was scared of it. I didn't want people to think I was starving myself. I didn't want to harm my body in any way. I began studying on the effects of longer fasts. after I had tried all the other methods. I wanted the best benefit for my body.

I had read that there is no benefit for having your fast days side-by-side, so I assumed that was true. Perhaps for some it is true, but for me, it has huge benefits as well. After doing intermittent fasting, and getting my body used to it for the last three years, I felt it was time to experiment with longer fasts.

I would do something that I call wraparound fasts. That's my own creation. I should patent it. Basically all I would do was extend the 5:2 Fast a little bit each time. For example, Monday I would not eat anything all day, and only drink water right through the evening until I went to bed. I started experimenting with extending that fast right up till noon the following day. I saw huge benefits in not only my weight, but the amount of fat that was burned. I quickly saw the spare tires around my waist disappear, little by little.

I do variations of my long fasts, or my wraparound fasts. Some days I do Wednesday-Thursday, some days I do Monday-Tuesday. Sometimes I do 24 hours back to back. Some days I do 16 hours back to back. I just play around with it and I always look forward to eating when I'm done. I love food, and I love it even more after I fast. You gain a new appreciation of everything you eat, and things taste much better as well.

I also don't crave sugar like I used to, but I've found that I really can eat anything I want now. Once your body retrains itself to burning fat instead of sugar for fuel, your metabolism changes back to what it was when you were a teenager. You can once again eat basically anything, and your body will tolerate it. Now, I wouldn't go overboard with this. You still want to eat healthy for maximum health benefits. I do this, but I also don't kick my butt if I have the occasional hamburger or treat.

One last thing I wanted to touch on, is one week fasts. I found some wonderful information about studies done, that show if you fast for five days, you can actually heal your immune system. It's wonderful research, especially for those who have gone through cancer treatments, and now find their immune system compromised. Fasting will literally rebuild it from scratch.

I tried my first weeklong fast at the end of the summer. I overindulged a little with too many barbecues and ice cream cones, so I felt I needed a good fast. Not that I put on any weight from my summer indulgence, but I felt it was a good time to do a weeklong fast, to give my body a better immune system, heading into the cold and flu season.

I started my fast on Monday, and only drank water straight through to Friday. I broke my fast on Saturday morning. I had no issues whatsoever, and it was the easiest thing I had ever done. I didn't feel hungry, and I had a boost of energy. People think that when you fast, you become week, but that is not the case at all. In fact, your body feels more energized. During my fast, I could think more clearly, handle stress better, and get more work done. It was so amazing, I am now going to do what I call, my immune boosting fast, every six months, to rebuild my immune system and fix whatever might be broken.

In conclusion to this chapter, I just wanted to give you a list of benefits to intermittent fasting. These have all been studied and proven:

- weight loss
- cellular repair
- increases human growth hormone and lengthens telomeres (little caps on your chromosomes that control how fast you age) The shorter the telomere, the faster you age. IF has been proven to lengthen telomeres, and reverses the effects of aging, and even in some instances, prevents aging.
- improves insulin levels
- lowers risk of type II diabetes
- helps you handle stress
- boosts energy
- prevents cancer
- rebuilds your immune system

- mental clarity
- prevents Alzheimer's
- helps to live longer
- brings back youthful glow
- fights wrinkles
- heals the gut

There are still so many things that I would love to tell you about intermittent fasting, that I just can't fit in this book. The benefits are endless. I would encourage you, especially those in menopause, to look into intermittent fasting. It will literally change your life. It did for me.

Chapter 7 – Editor's Pick

I wanted to make this chapter simple and list my regime, and the supplements that I take. Here is a list of my favorites that I use every day:

- Turmeric - Golden paste
- Vitex
- B-12
- B 100
- Cod Liver Oil
- Magnesium Bisglycinate
- Magnesium oil (my own recipe)
- Epson salt
- Coconut oil
- Zinc baby bum cream
- Kombucha tea (my own recipe)
- Pink Himalayan Salt
- Molasses

This is my daily natural therapy for menopause.

Conclusion

In conclusion, I just want to let you know that you don't have to let menopause destroy you. You don't have to let menopause rob you of your youth and beauty. It may be a huge change, but it doesn't have to be a negative one.

I used to think that women in menopause were old wrinkled has-beens. I used to think that the term menopause was reserved for those women with gray straggly hair and mustaches. I used to think menopause meant that you were somehow not female anymore, and your physical appearance was more manly than womanly.

All my preconceived ideas of menopause were wrong. It doesn't have to be this way. You don't have to fear losing your femininity. You don't have to accept weight gain. You don't have to get use to that spare tire. You don't have to have gray hair and manly qualities. You can fight this!

There is a difference between fighting it, and hating it. To hate it, means we are constantly thinking negatively toward menopause. I don't want you to do that. I want you to think positively toward menopause; to embrace it. If we carry those negative feelings, no good will come. Our bodies will not thrive under negative emotions. I found this to be true for my own self. If I constantly grumble about menopause, and the changes I see happening, I'm always down. Depression becomes huge, and I stumble with my self-esteem and body image. Brain chemistry changes when we're negative also, causing adverse health issues. I didn't want that, so I switched my perspective.

When I use the term *fighting it*, I am referring to that negative attitude toward menopause. You know, the one that tells you your life is over. That one that tells you you're going to be big and fat forever, so you might as well get used to it. That one that tells you you're never going to be healthy. That one that accepts the negative part of menopause. I didn't want to accept that, and I don't want you to accept that either. This is what I mean. Ladies, we have to fight it!

You can get back what you lost! You don't have to settle for obesity, or an unhealthy body, no matter what age you are, or what life changes you are going through. That is a lie. All it takes is a mind discipline. If we discipline our minds to look differently at menopause, we are already halfway there. My gynecologist was right when he said, "Welcome to your new life"

It *is* a new life, so embrace it! Try some natural remedies. Feel good! Let the sun shine in your life again. It's not too late just because you've hit menopause. You are beautiful! You are an amazing seasoned woman!

It's time to re-invent the new you!

The End

ABOUT THE AUTHOR

Kathleen Morris is the published author of numerous fiction and non-fiction books. She writes from the heart, and loves to empower women through research, information, and experience. When she's not writing, she's sewing, spending time with her family, or dreaming up her next project.